Never, Ever Give Up
Compiled by Allison Hite

© 2020 by Never, Ever Give Up CLE

ISBN: 978-1-950843-22-0

NEVER,
EVER
GIVE
UP

Anonymous Stories and Letters
from Northeast Ohio

To the wonderful and resilient people of Northeast Ohio. Your ability to create light, even in the darkest of times will continue to inspire more people than you can imagine. Thank you for sharing.

Never, Ever Give Up - CLE is a community project that asks folks in Northeast Ohio to write down one-page, anonymous stories all answering the question: What is the hardest thing you ever had to do?

Everyone has a story, and sharing our stories may be the most important thing we do for ourselves and for others. When we share our stories about hard times, we expose that we all have brokenness. It is not equal, but we all have it, and that is what connects us.

It can be hard to share stories that expose our pain and struggles, but sharing is a form of bravery. It gives the writer a chance to find their voice, recognize just how strong they are, and get some of the weight off their shoulders. We have to tell the truth in order to heal.

In response to these stories, Never, Ever Give Up - CLE collects Letters of Hope. These anonymous letters of encouragement, support, and connection help our writers feel seen and supported. Sometimes it can be hard to think of what to say when people share their pain. Often, we are scared to hurt the person even more by saying the wrong thing, but we must acknowledge what happened. Going through hard times can feel like a walk alone, but the act of bearing witness to the pain of others creates community. If the burden is left solely on the individual it can become too much to carry.

Never, Ever Give Up – CLE created a public installation at Hart Crane Park in Cleveland, OH from June 1, 2019 - August 31, 2019. The installation consisted of 130 stories and a five-foot tall yellow mailbox to collect Letters of Hope. A physical space for people to bear witness, build community, and honor resilience. This book is an extension of our time at Hart Crane Park.

To learn more visit:
NeverEverGiveUpCLE.com or
@NeverEverGiveUpCLE on Instagram.

The hardest thing I ever had to do was hug my friends mom at his wake after he took his own life.

I was very close with him in high school and his mom was one of the kindest women I had ever met. Once college started, we were still close but certainly did not talk as much.

Seeing his mom that day, I could not help but regret allowing our friendship to become more distant and not knowing he was hurting.

His mom told me she loved me, and through this experience, I learned to live life with more care. Tell people you care about them, because life is too short.

TO THE PERSON WHO HUGGED THEIR FRIEND'S MOM AT THE WAKE... A YEAR AGO A FRIEND OF MINE TOOK HIS LIFE AND HIS WAKE AND FUNERAL SERVICES WERE VERY EMOTIONAL AND MY HEAD WAS SWIMMING, THINKING OF HIM, HIS FAMILY, HIS WIFE, THE COMMUNITY HE HAD TOUCHED. IT WAS A SCARY AND UNEASY TIME IN MY MIND. I HUGGED EVERYONE I COULD AND SIMILARLY FOUND MYSELF EMBRACING THE BREVITY OF LIFE AND THE IMPORTANCE OF JUST BEING THERE FOR PEOPLE. EVERYONE NEEDS SOMEONE TO HUG. ♥

The hardest thing I've ever had to do was to begin taking Prozac for my mental health. I had been experiencing bouts of depression and anxiety while smiling in the faces of others. I had been skeptical about antidepressants, but figured that I needed to do what was right for me.

However, my parents were unaware and I was afraid of what they would think. I kept this from them for a month; only my friends at college knew. I felt kind of ashamed to be on Prozac, let alone have depression. Eventually, my counselor encouraged me to tell my parents. So, on Easter weekend when they came to visit, I finally told them and how I had _truly_ been feeling. They were completely understanding and immediately gave me their support. The best part of all? Knowing that I made a big step in my mental health journey.

To the person that said they had to take Prozac to help deal with their depression: Good for you! Way to face your fears about not being accepted by others, especially your parents, and for doing the right thing for your health. Some people may look down at you because of the stigma around mental health, but I am PROUD OF YOU! It takes a lot of grit to do something you are a little unsure about. Congratulations for telling your parents about your decision and standing up for yourself. NOW that they know, your journey towards well being is that much closer! Expanding your support group will allow you to know that everyone believes in you! I hope this letter helps you throughout your journey, however long that may be. Stay strong, and remember that YOU matter and that YOU ARE AMAZING!

Sincerely,
Your friend!

The hardest thing I ever had to do was take care of a sick baby at the age of 19. By 4 weeks old he was spitting up a lot and it even stopped his breathing a couple times. He was put on 2 different medications that had to be timed with his feedings and a monitor for his breathing. At 12 weeks he was projectile vomiting and his pediatrician thought I was some dumb kid and wouldn't listen. I trusted my gut and took him to a different doctor. A week later my 3 month old baby was having surgery. I learned to trust my gut and motherly instincts and even though I was young my love for my son was enough in that moment to get him the proper care.

On July 29 2018, my older sister, along with her boyfriend and 2 others, were killed in an ISIS terrorist attack in Tajikistan; life since July 29 2018 has been the most difficult and painful thing I have had to go through and will continue to go through for the rest of my life. Since July 29, 2018, I have relapsed with drinking, relapsed with an eating disorder that caused me to go below 95 pounds, and have been overwhelmed with severe depression and anxiety; I was angry at the world and universe for my older sister being taken away. However, on December 1st, I came to the realization that I was making the situation worse with my coping mechanisms and anger. Yes, it is ok to be angry, and I know my older sister would understand my anger and frustration, but, my sister, such a bright and positive soul, would want me, as well as everyone she knew, to see the positives and beauty in each and every day. With all this said, I now have several months of sobriety under my belt with the help of family, friends, Sober Grid, and Smart Recovery, I now am 120 pounds and have a healthier relationship with food and exercise thanks to the help of a nutritionist, and I have been seeing a psychiatrist to help manage my depression and anxiety. If there is one piece of wisdom I can give, it is that no matter what life throws at you, things will get better; stay positive, surround yourself with supportive, encouraging, and loving people, and obtain help when you need it. #NEVERGiveUP

I was living in a foreign country and had been sexually assaulted. I was terrified of telling anyone, and when I finally did, I was shamed and told that it was probably my fault. I was shocked! I felt not only violated, but also betrayed, alone, and stuck.

When I came back to the U.S., I didn't tell my family at first and tried desperately to get back to a normal routine. Weeks later, when I started experiencing symptoms of **PTSD**, I had no idea what was wrong with me. I hated myself and thought I was crazy! I couldn't sleep and felt more anxiety than I had ever felt in my life. My friends + family didn't understand.

Finally, I decided to seek help through counseling. I still was not able to connect the dots from my assault to my **PTSD**, nor did I know at the time that that was what I was experiencing; I just knew I needed help. I remember trembling while sitting in my car during my lunch break to call and make an appointment. I felt so scared and vulnerable. I'M so glad I was brave and made the call.

I've been on this healing journey for almost 10 years and there are still so many hard things. I'm still really angry that this happened to me, and angry that I have to do so much work to heal. I don't know if my anger will ever subside, but I know now that that's ok too. I'M thankful for the support I've received and have learned that we humans are incredibly resilient and I know that I really am so strong. Healing is not a straight path, but I'm learning to be gentle with myself, and I'm really glad for that. ♥

Having gone through
hard stuff is not
shameful, it is

HUMAN

Thanks for sharing ♡

The hardest thing I've ever had to do was to have the responsibility to tell medical staff to remove my 4 month old daughter, Remi, from the respirator that maintained her breathing. It wasn't that actual directive to the staff to take her off that breathing machine; it was the internal negotiation that I had to come to terms with that proved hardest. The hospital had, on a previous emergency visit, suggested that things would not get better for her; that her breathing would stop more and more frequently and that I was welcomed to leave her at the hospital and walk away. They were my enemies in my post partum defense mode state of being. But I had to seek inside myself that center where love and reality co-exist. I had to do what was best for her. I had to let her go. I gave my consent.

To the parent of sweet little Remi,
your courage is boundless for the
choice you made. Sometimes, I blurt
out to God, "Why? Why would anyone
need to go through something like that?"
I hope you find ease + peace in your
heart and know that I see you. ♡
Sending endless love your way
to your courageous heart.

Getting over a break-up with the person I considered my soul-mate was one of thee hardest endeavors I had to overcome. It took a long time to heal from it, I'm still healing to this day. The way that I had to Get over it was to one. accept responsibility, two. embrace the Pain / the situation, 3. reflect and 4. do what I love to do most in the world..... write.

peace

To the person who broke up with their soulmate. Its such a difficult situation to realize the person you were involved with no longer shares the same goals, path, desires + love that you do. We all change + the hope is to grow + change together. I recently made the decision to leave my spouse of 12years while working to raise 2 children. I am afraid of what the future holds but I know that I have begun my journey on the path that will bring me + my children happiness for the life we are living now. The power of positivity, kindness + compassion for myself will continue to guide me throughout as I hope it guides you. ☮💗

The hardest thing I had
to do was decide to live
after overdosing on my
medication. On May 31,
2017 a good friend of
mine died by suicide.
I was filled with
survivor guilt. I missed
him tremendously. In
July I had the idea that
if I died I could be with
him again. I lived through
my suicide attempt and
instead of trying again
I decided to seek help. I
still miss him every
single day and I am
coming upon the two
year anniversary, but
at least I can discuss
my grief with my therapist

To: The hardest thing I had to do was decide to live after overdosing...

ABOUT ONE MONTH AGO I LOST MY NEPHEW TO SUICIDE. HE HAD SUFFERED FROM DEPRESSION FOR MANY YEARS AND IT EVENTUALLY COST HIM HIS LIFE. I WAS THERE THE DAY HE WAS BORN AND UNFORTUNATELY I WAS THE ONE THAT HAD TO TELL MY SISTER HE HAD DIED. I WISH I WOULD HAVE BEEN ABLE TO HAVE ONE MORE CONVERSATION, ONE MORE HUG, ONE MORE TEXT SO I'LL TELL YOU — YOU ARE AN AMAZING PERSON, YOU ARE LOVED, YOU ARE RIGHT THAT LIFE ISN'T FAIR AND IT'S VERY TOUGH AT TIMES. I THINK YOU HAVE MADE AN INCREDIBLE CHANGE IN YOUR LIFE AND I'M SO GRATEFUL YOU ARE STILL ON EARTH WITH ME. ADMITTING YOU NEEDED HELP AND SEEKING IT OUT WAS A HUGE STEP AND IM SO PROUD OF YOU! TAKE ONE DAY AT A TIME, TAKE TIME TO BE THANKFUL FOR THINGS IN YOUR LIFE — LARGE AND SMALL. AS YOU AND I BOTH KNOW LIFE IS PRECIOUS SO LIVE EACH MOMENT AND LET THOSE AROUND KNOW YOU LOVE THEM. I'M PROUD OF YOU AND GLAD I WAS ABLE TO WRITE YOU THIS NOTE. FROM ONE STRANGER TO ANOTHER

THE HARDEST THING I EVER HAD TO DO IS BELIEVE IN MYSELF. EVERY DAY I HAVE TO REMIND MYSELF THAT MY VOICE MATTERS AND THAT MY IDEAS HAVE MERIT. THE DAILY WAVES OF NEGATIVITY MAKES ME WANT TO QUIT. BUT I TELL MYSELF I WANT TO BE HAPPY.

To the person who wrote "The hardest thing
I ever had to do is believe in myself".
Your voice does matter and so do your ideas.
Keep believing in yourself no matter what
negativity comes your way. You are
stronger than you will ever realize.
In moments of doubt think of the
qualities you have that you are grateful
for. Happiness is found within. Keep
believing and you will keep being
happy. I reacted to your story and am
sending you words of wisdom because
I also am having a hard time believing
in myself. I keep getting denied job interview
after job interview and the hardship
sometimes makes me not believe in
myself. You are not alone. Believing is
succeeding.

The hardest thing I ever had to do
was fix myself when I was broken.
I have Suffered with a series of
Things... depression, anxiety, bulimia
and anorexia. I first noticed I had
an actual problem when my best
friend's mom hugged me saying how
thin I got. At my lightest I was
86 pounds, normally I'm around
130. During that time I was in an
abusive relationship, and was being
told by him and everyone I cared
about that I wasn't good enough.
I still Struggle but years later
it has gotten better. With time
everything gets better, with love and
Support, it gets better... without my
best friend's mom worrying about me
I'm not sure where I would be but I
do know that she helped me
fix myself when I was broken.

Recover from an
eating disorder
without the help of my
mom.
She's aware now, and
she's very supportive.
I just wish I hadnt
been afraid to tell her
before.

To the person who had to recover from an eating disorder without her mom i understand. some of my loved ones went through the same thing. I was there for them when their parents werent. I know now hard it is to experience that when you think that your own mom doesnt even care or understand. Filling in for the role of a mother was difficult but she knew i was always there.

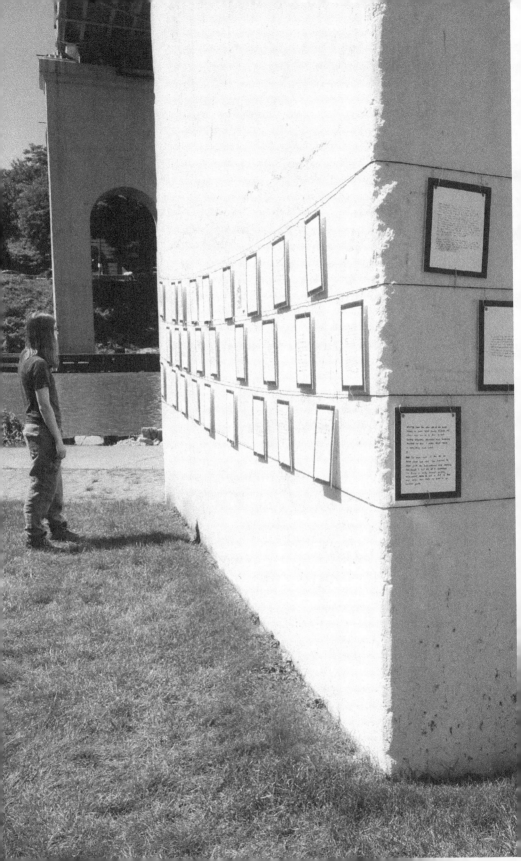

The hardest thing I have ever had to do was say goodbye to my dog. I know that it might sound not that bad to some people but, this dog was with me when my mom went through a rare form of breast cancer, this dog was with me when my parents got divorced and my mom was a single mom taking care of six kids. this dog was always here for <u>everything</u> and he was really my bestfriend. He was also here when my sister was in the hospital because they couldn't figure out why she was sick, he was here when I found out that my little brother wasn't the same as everyone else, and thing that I have no problem doing because he is mentally challenged. But he was always here to support me and love me no matter what.

To the person who said goodbye
to their dog—

Our animals are with us and love
us unconditionally their whole lives.
It is not easy to say goodbye
and it leaves a hole in our lives.
Don't let anyone tell you that it's
not that bad.

I recently lost my dog too and I
still get sad about it. The days
get easier as you build new routines.
I like to focus on my good memories
of him and how grateful I am for
his love through the years.
I hope that your hurt dulls and
that you know how lucky you are
to have had such an amazing
friend.

The Hardest Thing I've Ever Had to Do...
was grieve my mother's death. My
mother + I were not close. She had
multiple mental health issues which
got in the way of her mothering. And
I spent years in therapy untangling
all that had happened to me in my
childhood. One key moment was when
I said to my therapist "I'm going to
miss my mother when she dies - and
I never thought I'd ever say that."
And that was indeed the Truth when that
time came. I did miss her. And I
missed all the tenderness + love that I
never received from her - or gave.
    My grief was full-blown, raw,
painful. And yet I walked through
it, moment by moment. I cried, I talked
to others, I journaled - I paid attention
to my internal landscape. I gave
myself over to what was moving
through me. I persevered. I took things
a day at a time. I opened myself to
the love I had missed, but now found within.

The hardest thing I've ever had to do was survive being shot in a drive by. I had/have to overcome the look of fear on my son's face as bullets flew past his head. I've learned to forgive the man ~~you~~ who made a bad choice and almost took my life and my son's. Beyond the physical pain and trauma, I've had to learn to love people who ~~are~~ are the hardest to love because they need love the most.

The hardest thing I ever had to do was realize that I do not need to please everyone. Until recently, I felt like I had to agree with everyone, get along with everyone, and do things I did not want to do to avoid conflict. I was putting my own needs, desires, & GOALS aside. As a result, I found myself in miserable relationships & friendships that were completely wrong for me. I was never truly happy and spent so much time feeling this way. Then, due to an extremely tough and personal circumstance (one of those situations that ends up teaching an important lesson), I found myself. Yes, as cliché as that sounds. I realized that I can live my life the way I want to live it. I have found true friends & begun living a life more extraordinary than I could have ever imagined. I have never been so STRONG.

I spent a week in a single room with my then gf. With her being over 300 miles away, I thought I had everything I could ask for right in front of me. I got a call Saturday afternoon from my mother, who said she felt something was off. She felt there was something I was keeping from her. "Are you pregnant?" "Are you depressed?" "Are you gay?" I choked. I cried. My heart pounded. It took every bit of courage for me to muster a simple yes. My gf ran to the next room upon hearing our conversation, knowing my very traditional, Christian mother wouldn't respond well. This was the day I came out to my mother. She cut me off for a few months after, but eventually it got better. Although this was the hardest thing I've done, it was the most rewarding.

This was the day I finally became myself.

The hardest thing I've ever had to do is get through College. During those 4 long years I spend alot of time on an emotional roller coaster. My good times were really good and my bad times were really really bad. As an 18yr old black girl in a new town I felt very alone, undeserving, and insecure. During these time I was challenged not only academically, but emotionally as well. I had to learn to not only humble my self and ask for help but to accept and begin to love myself. After many failed exams, failed relationships, and new hair cuts and colors I made it to Senior year. I had come close to dropping out 3 different times due to financial reasons, mental health issues, and academic struggles. However I made it. I persevered by assuring myself I can do this. In my worst times, crying in my bed I kept pushing myself by saying I can do this. I thought about all my siblings who were looking up to me, my mom who was so proud of me, and my community that was counting on me. The love for my family and their love for me is what got me through my hardest time. ♥
#firstgen #blackgirlmagic #DONTQUIT

To all of those who shared
their stories of courage, faith
and perserverance —

    I see you
    I hear you
    I honor your strength
    I will help support you

The hardest thing I have had to do is watch my grandfather succumb to Alzheimer's. I spent an extraordinary amount of time with them when I was young and other than my parents and sister, I don't think anyone had a bigger effect on me than he did. After elementary school, our family started noticing changes in him. Over the course of ten years his personality, memory and physical health slowly but surely deteriorated. It seemed unfair because he was the most spirited, joyful and playful person in my life. He was also the best story teller. It was hard to see the effects it had on my grandma and mom. It aged them and slowly broke their hearts.

Luckily, I spent enough time with him when he was "himself" to remember him that way. And I try to honor his memory by not taking life too seriously, for making time for sharing stories, and approaching life with an adventurous optimism to facilitate having experiences that are worth sharing. And when I'm facing a seemingly relentless string of challenges or bad days I remember how steadfast my mom and granma were in caring for someone they loved, year after year

34

So, I'm writing this in relation to your grandfather having Alzheimers. I actually work at a nursing home on that unit specifically. I've seen the effects it has on not only my residents but their family. You are a STRONG individual and I hope you continue to not ^let this affect to the point you're not able to keep your head up. Just know, there is always someone around you who, not only understands, but will be there for you without hesitation. ♥

· I remember other parts of it like it was yesterday, some better than others. No one really thinks that it will happen to them, that it only happens to other people or in movies/tv. But I can tell you it happened to me. He was my friend, one I actually had a crush one. All it was supposed to be was his kind gesture of walking me back to my dorm. I was just wearing a tank top and shorts. Fast forward several hours. I had just been raped by someone I cared about. I was curled up in a ball crying. so scared and shut down. I didn't fully understand what had happened until I was on an exam table at the ER getting a rape kit, done. I got it done but didn't report... I was scared of what people would say and how they would react. someone even said, "are you sure that's what happened?, You should feel lucky a guy would like you"

· If I could I go back I would've pressed charges, he needs to know what he did wasn't ok.

36

To the person who was raped,
you are right - what he did
was NOT okay. No matter
who you are, what the
situation is, what you were
wearing - never okay. I'm so
sorry you have to carry this
now. I believe you. I can't
wait to see you shine again.

The hardest thing I have ever done is watch my son destroy his beautiful, creative life with addiction. I hope he has started to heal. ♡

To the person who had to watch their son battle with addiction, I'm so sorry you had to go through that. I must be so difficult for you to watch him do that to himself. I think you should let him know that you're there for him, and tell him how you feel about his addiction. I think If you two try to help each other, than you will both benefit.

Its very difficult for anyone to watch some they care about battle addiction, but its espicaily hard for a mother to watch her child go through something as horrible as that. I think you should know, its nothing you could have stopped, and there was no way for you to prevent it. Its not your fault. There's always options for therapy and theres always people for you to talk to it you need to talk. Stay strong!

♡

The hardest thing I had to do and still have to do is face the fact that I put on a fake smile and pretend everything is ok. the truth is that I have so much anxiety and lack of confidence. I constantly compare myself to others and can't stop myself. I only see the negative and can't fall asleep. my mind is always busy thinking about the worst Possibility. I also never tell anyone how I feel. I'm scared. I feel like no one will believe me. There are people out there with bigger problems that I seem small and so do my problems. I listen to what other people say and let it get the best of me. I have image issues, but the only response I get when I tell People is OMG no you are gorgeous. or your so skinny when I know inside I feel the opposite and look the opposite. I try everyday to find the positive, but never comes. someday it will get better.

To the person who wrote about putting on a fake smile, I understand what that's like. Through most of high school, I put on a facade of who I thought others expected me to be. I wasn't confident in myself, and suffered from anxiety and depression. It was a perpetual sadness, but like you, the thing that kept me going was the thought that things would be different one day. Now, I'm still working on taking care of myself, but I know I can get through this because of those going through the same thing we are. I wish you only the best. We can get through this together. ♡

I had to ride with out
traing wheels too it was
hard   and frustrated
but   it well be fine
I got it to but it
well   pay off it will
be   better then with
no   traing wheels. you can
ride in the grass! So it
is easy to get aound cars!

42

TO the girl who's hardest thing
was learning how to ride a bike.
You are not alone I didn't learn
how to ride a bike until I was 9
years old. I felt left out with all
my friends who could ride bikes.
It is okay, because it is hard but
you can get through it. It can
be embarressing, but you will
get through it ♥

The hardest thing I ever had to do was overcome my fear of speaking in public. I faced it by practicing speaking in front of my family and when the time came, I did great. And I haven't had that much of a problem since

To the person who wrote about their fear
of public speaking:

I also used to have a fear of public speaking!
And it was inconvenient, because I like to
do theatre. Fortunately, I got over it eventually.
And you did too, it seems! Good for you!
But don't ever be embarassed by being nervous
about it. Chances are, everyone you're speaking
in front of is also nervous!

Good luck with your future speaking

The hardest thing I ever had to do was Perserver thourgh my grand father dying in a car accident whie I was in the hospital because I had an stomach virus I was crying because of both reasons but I was also sad a month later I went to his funeral I was crying hard I had to perserver by doing arts and crafts also playing basketball with my cousions but it was hard because me and him use to do the same things together.

To the person who wrote about their grandfather
passing while in the hospital...

It's amazing to hear how you used art and
other things to help get through your
loss. Your grandfather would be so happy you
continued doing those things. Never give
that up and know that you're always
surrounded by love!

Moving from the other side of the world.
Having to leave some family, friends, and
places that are all so dear to me.
Getting extremely depressed and homesick
because all that I could think about
is everything back home.

♡

(And) I've been here in the US for
three years now and I've learned to
move past the homesickness and sadness
even though I feel bits of it sometimes.
I've found a lovely second family,
heavensent ~~from~~ ~~(a)~~ and so full of love
and care. They help me even in my
hardest parts.

To the person who moved halfway across the world,

Your courage is amazing.. Like you said, the move wasn't easy, but you have perservered and you are still here, and for that, I applaud you. I'm sure the choice was not easy, but when your hope falters, remember why you chose to move. All those reasons and motivations are still there to remind you that you made the right choice for you. Someday, I hope I can be as brave as you and move somewhere new.

You are amazing

THERE IS HOPE

The hardest part in my life that
I remember was when I
cheated in science class for
a test, I was at school it
was time to switch, my class
went next door, we did the
the test. ~~before~~ While i was
doing my test i remembered
the practice text, then i
pulled it out and coppied
it. I got in trouble. A few
weeks later i told my
Mom and it was OK.

To the person that got caught cheating
on a test, try and learn from your mistake.
Next time you have a test, study hard during
that week so you feel confident you will do good.
It is okay to make a mistake, but try not
to repeat the mistake. As humans, we
aren't perfect and we constantly make mistakes
and do immoral things. All we can do is
change and grow.

The hardest I've had to do was to take a toxic friend out of my life. It was only hard because I still cared for them even though they were toxic, only cared for themself, and made me feel less than them. I still loved them & wanted them to be my best friend. Even though I didn't need them.

To the person who had to cut their friend out of their life. There is nothing wrong with cutting a toxic relationship out of your life. As these toxic relationships can only have a bad affect on us, and will stop us from doing that we want in life or stop us from growing or whatever it may be. I am feeling this right now as one of my friends brings out he worst in me and we tend to not get along. Reading your story gave me more courage to cut my friend off as it isn't good for me. It is good for us to me selfish sometimes, especially in these situations. So I am proud of you for doing the right thing and hope you are doing great ☺

The hardest thing I've ever had to do is grow up. Over these years, I've been running through the obstacle course of life. I saw it got hard, and the longer I ran, the more I grew. I was so scared and angry that I had to grow. I wanted to stay young forever. Later in life, on this obstacle course, I met two people who vowed to grow up with me, by my side. We grew up, but we made it good, we made growing up, happier. I realized that growing up isn't as sad as. I thought. I am still growing, and I'm happy. I am living.

To the ~~person~~ person who had to grow up,

I promise growing up is worthit.
you **will** meet so many good
people and have so many great
experiences. Growing up will be hard,
it will suck sometimes. But people
are always gonna be by your
side,

Signed,

a person
who grew up.

The hardest thing I ever had to do was admit that I was powerless over drugs and alcohol. I was ruining my life and the lives of the people I cared about most, but I didn't want to get help. I didn't care whether I lived or died... Now, I DO care and I'm so glad I made that first step. To anyone who is reading this and struggling with addiction, you are not alone. You are loved. There is

HOPE.

o the person who wrote about being powerless to drugs and alcohol, I salute you. Addiction is something that lots of people n my family struggle with, It's extremely hard to go through but it is not your fault. You are so brave for telling your story and just know that there is always someone there for you.

The hardest battle I ever fought, was beating an opiate addiction. I used drugs for 10 years of my short life.

In Recovery, I have 4 years sober, started my own family & have the most loving partner a person could ask for

There is hope ♡

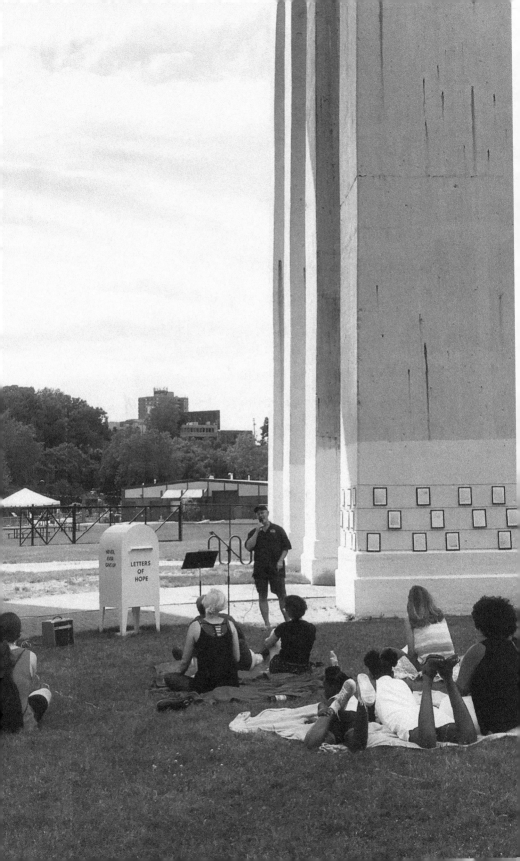

The hardest thing I ever did was
move to a new country at the
age of 12 without knowing the
language, culture or people!

I overcame it by through the help of my
parents, and by focusing on the task ahead of me.

"Don't put it in pack, with miles to go;
need a matchs, nevermore shall we read in
the dark"

To the person who wrote about moving
to a new country at 12 years old,
I'm inspired by your bravery!
What you did at 12 years old is
harder than what many people do
throughout their lives. I moved to
a new state when I was 13, and
even that transition was hard. I can't
begin to understand the difficulties
you've overcome. Your story of
resilience and determination will
give hope to so many. I hope
that you are proud of what you
have already accomplished, and
confident in what you can achiev
moving forward.

YOU ARE A HERO

I have a disability a learn disability read and write is hard. But I really want to be a auther and have my book publish. I didn't have the money or any way. One day someone told me about self- publish. I look in to it. And ~~went~~ then I did

I made a few mistakes a long the way but I finally did it and I'm still going strong

P. S. When you read this if there something you really want to do, do it.

No matter what people say or disadvantage you may have good Luck 🙂

To the person who wants to write but has a hard time due to a disability: The only way to overcome a challenge is through determination and courage. If you keep working at this challenge and never give up, You can reach this goal and overcome this obstacle through persistence. Have faith in your ability to write and always strive to do your best in whatever you do. I believe that you can do whatever your heart desires as long as you keep working towards it

HARDEST thing to
Do is being a single
Black, INtelligent feMAle.

Letter of Hope

To the single, Black, intelligent female...

Continue being the best you. ~~XXXXXX~~

You are worth it.

We are worth it.

Stand in your power.

TO THE SINGLE BLACK INTELLIGENT
FEMALE...

IT MAY BE THE HARDEST BUT
IT ALSO MAKES YOU THE
AWESOMEST. KEEP ON BEING
STRONG FOR ALL OF US

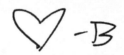 -B

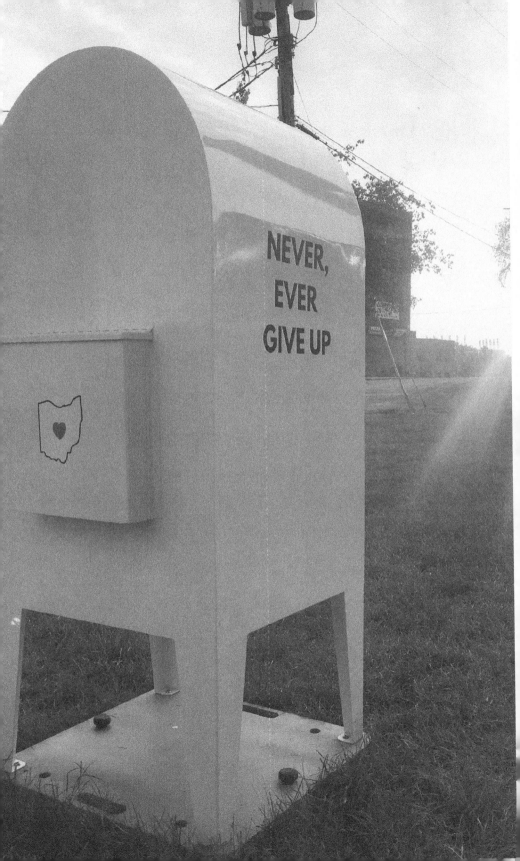

The hardest thing I've ever done is Realize that I needed to fix myself and ask for the help to do that.

I have struggled with depression most of my life. I hit a low in 2015-2016. I was getting divorced and living a state away from my newborn daughter. Therapy wasn't helping enough + I contemplated ending it.

I asked friends, family, + co-workers for help. I got medication + started researching & experimenting with my health. I listened to other people's struggles and advice.

I made changes, cut out toxic people, and brought in good people. I now have a wonderful group of supportive people, a positive relationship with my daughter, and for the first time in years some real hope about my future.

To the person who wrote about asking for help to fix yourself:

Thank you. One of the strongest and most courageous acts a person can do is recognize when help is needed and taking the steps to ACTUALLY find that help. YOU are the reason the idea of seeking guidance with depression, anxiety, and any personal obstacles is becoming more accepted and less stigmatized

I am inspired by your abilities to take the necessary steps to reduce the negative and increase the positive in your life. Because you DESERVE it. Everybody does.

I hope you have found and continue to find happiness, peace, and joy in your life that you genuinely deserve.

The hardest thing in life I ever had to do...
Walk away from my psychologically & emotionally
Abusive husBAND who was Dying of cancer.
The abuse escillated to physical abuse
as he left me STRANDED 500 miles away from home.
During his good days after chemo, he
would spend his good days with other
people, not me. I was left to be the
nurse maid & chauffer. I decided to
get a Restraining order & made a plan
to escape while I filed for divorce
after 13 years; 12 aBusive. I embraced
my strength and left 11 months before
his death.

My children's father was abusive and a few times, he was abusive to my son. There are several reasons why the hardest thing I've had to do so far is devorce him. The main thing is I didn't want to cause my children any pain, but their father was causing them pain. I believed in the vows I took at my wedding. While married, I didn't work much, so I didn't have a good source of income. I didn't want my children's quality of life to change. It wasn't easy, but we got through it. My family and friends were a major help. They helped us with a place to live; assisted me in finding work and moral support as well. We went to counseling for a while, which helped us mentally. Most of all, my children were supportive and very well behaved.

One of the hardest things I have ever had to do was leaving an abusive relationship. I never thought I would be in that position, but it happened so fast and I was in love. I saw the signs, but I always made excuses. I told myself, "I know it's over, but I'll wait until X happens." Then X happened and I wouldn't leave.

Finally, there was a breaking point. My life was in shambles and he couldn't see that. So I ended things. It sucked, when I was already going through so much, but it helped in the end. I would still ask myself, "What if I stayed?" or "Maybe, It was me, not him?" And I hate that. But this isn't an hour and a half movie, so the hard things take time to deal with, and that is okay.

To the person who realized I am
someone, I do not have to go
through abuse:

I have seen in my life all forms of
abuse, I have realized those who
never faced abuse do not understand.
They say that will never be me or
anyone I know, I will never be an
abuser. I am here to tell you in a
world of I never met you I feel
your pain. You are somebody! You
have the right to continue on the
journey of self love and what is
truly the best for you in the
future. You are the voice of today
and tomorrow, you are the light
and joy of the world. You are
loved. If you would have stayed
in abuse, you would continue
the thought of this is what love
looks like and it is not! I am
here to tell you that the pain you
had is a testimony to realize
there was more in store for you.
Healing is a process and this
shall pass.

The hardest thing I have to get over is telling my mom that I am bisexual sometimes its hard for me to get it out some day im going to tell her ~~that~~ the day I tell her she wont be mad I just hope she reddy for what im going to tell her

Tell her on your own time...
And even if she doesn't
understand right away
it's okay. She's always
loved you exactly as you
are. Bisexuality included

the hardest thing I ever had to do
was watch my Dad suffer from
cancer and pass on from us. I watched
and witnessed my mom and brother
unravel and have their hearts
beaten, as I did the same. I did
not think it was possible a parent
would really die. It's impossible to
describe the darkness that follows,
even with the sharing of loving memories.
But we are all still here, we survived,
are working, and are fulfilling our lives
constantly thinking of my Dad and his
humble, kind, impeccably calm & generous
person we all share. There is hope in
surviving & giving back to everyone you meet
through their example ♡

The hardest thing I have ever had to do is say goodbye to my mom. Coming to that reality that my mom would no longer physically be here to be apart of life's happenings with me is still surreal in many moments. When my mom looked at me like she didn't want to leave me yet, not so soon; I saw the sadness in her eyes. I knew she'd been fighting as long as she could, but she was tired. I felt in my spirit that my grammy (my mom's mother) and my great-aunt (my mom's aunt) was telling her to come on and be with them in Heaven. The hardest thing that I had to do is be in the room with my mom in her final moments in this world. I held her hand and told her that I love her. The hardest thing has been and still to some point currently keeping it together on the outside while being broken on the inside; not knowing exactly how to express the grief. I know my mom is at peace because she knows Christ. It's just her not being here is a challenging life shift for me. I love you mom always and I hope that I am giving you a reason to smile from Heaven.

The hardest thing to do sometimes...
Moving forward

To anyone who wrote about loss...
The hardest thing I have
ever done is to hold my dad's
hand as he passed away. He
was a wonderful father, and full
of life until the very end. I
miss Mom and Dad so much.
I have hope that I can be
as good a parent that they
were. And I hope to love my
husband just as Mom and Dad
were devoted one to the other,
I hope you can feel that, too.

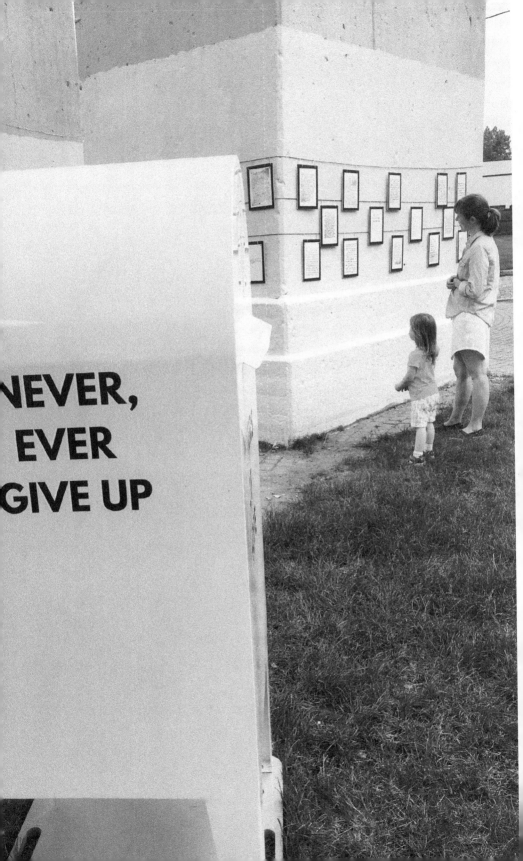

The hardest thing I've every had to do was, Love my self.

To the person that wrote about loving themsevles,

It's okay, we've all been there before. I have struggled
in the past with loving myself as well. It has brought
anxiety and increased self-awareness. I was struggling
so hard it was affecting my every day life, so I appreciate
you sharing your story. One day, I decided the only way
to beat this is to accept who I am and acknowledge I
am not perfect. I started to look at my flaws as unique
quirks just as I accepted my strengths. Over time, my self
image and confidence started seeing a positive twirl. I
encourage would everyone who is struggling to love themselves,
to recognize their flaws, and acknowledge that their flaws
are a part of them and that part makes them just as unique
as their strengths. ♡

The hardest thing I ever had to to do was for learn divison. When I first started learning divison It was really REALLY hard I had to do problems like 22÷2 or 36÷6 and I thought I could not do It. Then my 4th grade teacher tought me and I had got It all down and now I know how to do problems like 144÷12.

When I was a senior at Ohio State, I found out I was pregnant with my 1st son. :) Two days later my internship doors closed. This was a requirement for graduation :). At that time only available internships was located in dayton and cincinnati which was going to be a struggle due to me being in classes in columbus. Taking long drives back and forth, struggles with 1st trimester sickness I was determined to complete college for my unborn! HARDEST THING EVER NEVER, EVER GIVE UP!! :)

The hardest thing I ever had to do was cope with getting type one diabetes when I was 12. My life changed so quickly and I had no idea what was ahead. Even though it has been 11 years since I was first diagnosed, diabetes is still a struggle for me everyday. It is something that never goes away, no matter how hard I try to ignore that it is there. Something I'm still trying to figure out is how to balance it all. Even when I'm busy with something, I still have to deal with my diabetes.

Diabetes isn't all bad though. It has helped me realize how strong I am, and that I can pretty much get through anything that comes my way. Talking about my disease has helped me too. Since I've had problems confronting my illness, talking about it outloud has helped me come to terms with diabetes always being in my life.

The hardest thing is to learn English. Because the Pronounciation is not easy. But I will try my best.

我會努力的～.

The hardest thing I ever had to do was beat cancer! And I did!! I had to fight hard, to get through Chemotherapy, Radiation, and two surgeries. It was worth it, because I cherish life now. It was my wake-up call! Everything can change in one day. Beating cancer is brutal, and wears you out completely. At times, I felt the task was impossible, cruel, and never ending. Luckily, I had an army of family, friends, Doctors, and Nurses who fought with me, and prayed for me! Now, I am writing a book about cancer, filled with poetry, humor and tips. To all you Warriors out there, Never Give Up! You can do it! Reach out to someone — You are never alone!

The hardest thing I have ever done was deciding that I deserve to be happy. After struggling with depression and negative thoughts for so long, I finally told myself that I was worth more than the image I had painted of myself. I finally started taking care of myself. I took breaks when I needed to. I stopped being self-depreciating, even in humor. I connected to the people around me and found that they had so much love to give. And so do I. I wanted to give that love to the world. And through that, I connected even closer to those around me. In one particular case, very close.

That's not to say that the depression is gone. No matter how much you may wish for it, that never truly goes away. But if you can find the attitude to fight it, you just might find others who are willing to fight with you.

The Loss of my husband devistated me. He was my best friend and lover. He changed me and showed me how to be a better person. He taught me how not to be afraid of people and of life. But when he died I was Lost. I stopped taking care of myself. I have no direction. I'm so alone. But I know he wouldn't like that. So I am trying. Trying to do things - keep busy while still missing him. So I just have to keep Trying to get through every day. And forgive those who have not been supportive. But hopefully, if/when I Remember the love and the good memories - it will get me through. Love never dies. I hold on to that The love of my soul mate will last forever!

Everyone who wrote
these notes took
the first step.✱
Letting others help us —
And this shows we
are not alone.
We can all do this
together.
Some of us have
watched people die,
Some of us are
learning to Forgive,
others need to
make friends in a
New place.
But we can do
this —
Together

The hardest thing I ever had to do was lay my father to rest. He was very close to me and loved, nurtured, & cared for me since I could remember.

The second hardest decision I had to make is deciding to keep or abort my child. It was a decision to be made with logic over emotion. Emotionally I felt heartbroken to ever even think of not keeping my child. But logically I thought about how hard it would be for me to support my child, mentally, emotionally, finacially, etc. With both me & the childs father being full time students trying to better ourselves I came to conclusion it wasn't the best decision to keep my child. I want the best for my children, so now I will keep working to get to that lifestyle to be able to support my future children.

To the person that wrote about
losing their father, and then struggling
later in life with the decision to
get an abortion or not. You've been
through so much, I hope you see how
strong you are. I certainly do! I think
that it's wonderful that you want to
wait until the conditions are right for
you to have a child. You deserve to feel
ready when/if that happens!

You are such an empowered woman,
and your dad would be proud of
everything you are.

You are loved!!

warmly,

your friend :)

The hardest thing I ever had to do was, watch my life fall apart right in front of my eyes. I literally invested everything into a relationship with someone who used me, mentally, sometimes physically, emotionally abused me. I had my car repoed, I was evicted from my apartment, and my credit was in the water all at the age of 19. Prior to learning about adulthood so early in life, I went through even more as a kid, about 7-9 years old. I watched my dad grow as an alcoholic, and my mom be physically and mentally/emotionally abused by him. My closest grandparents passed away in the mist of all this and things just got worse. Ultimately my parents gave up on each other. Me & my moms bond become unpatchable. She blamed me for my Father and all the other hardships she experienced after having me. Then the guy she almost married (my step dad), first closest feeling of having a father figure, was murdered on the west side of Cleveland. Ever since a kid, I feel I've been on this never ending cycle of losses whether financially or emotionally. I just want more than anything to get my life together as well as boost my self esteem. I just don't know how because when I feel like Im doing good or right something happens to push me 30,000 steps back. Me and my parents bonds are horrible still, I Don't know what to do.

To the person who feels they take 20,000 steps back whenever it's finally going right in life:

You said that you didn't know what to do to cope in your letter. I wanted to let you know that you are already doing it. Being brave enough to reach out, let people know how you feel takes so much courage—much more than smiling & pretending everything is okay.

In all of our lives, we will continually get knocked down. Thats okay. Thats how we learn what we can handle. Being open, honest & willing to accept kindness will help each of us keep moving forward. And caught up in all the bad will be glimmers of good that help you remember why you keep getting up everyday—even when its hard & you dont know why you do.

I know it's a little cliché, but you are not alone. You've got this. And if you need advice, start by getting up every day for the people you love. Eventually, you'll be one of those people too & you'll be able to get up for yourself.

♡

The hardest thing I have had to conquer is the beast of depression. The voices in my head telling me I'll never get better, I'll measure upto the expectations in my head. Being dragged down time and time again into the abys of darkness gasping for air searching for light. In the 12 ~~suic~~ attempts I have taken to end my precious life the hardest thing I chose to do was live. Fight. Breath.

To the person who wrote about trying to attempt to take their own life 12 times... I am so sorry that that was what you felt was the only option, but I want you to know that although I do not know you, I know that you have a full life ahead of you. You have the ability to change your own life with every decision you make. You hold so much potential and the possibilities to what you can accomplish are endless. Just by sharing your story, you have taken an important step and you have affected me. I wish you the best of luck in the future and I am so proud of you.

I was diagnosed with cancer in my late 20's and went through a year of injecting some pretty crazy chemicals into my body. I'm someone who loves to live life & be active so resting in bed and recovery was really hard. I'm now 10+ cancer free & glad that year is behind me.

To the person who ~~battled~~ battled
cancer. I understand because my dad
had hodgkins desease which is a type of
cancer. He had 16 chemo treatments but
fought really hard and made it.
Keep trying and you'll acomplish anything
and win every battle

To the woman ~~fighting~~ who fought cancer in her
20's - while I have never gone through something
intense + hard as that, I have witnessed so many
people go through a similar cancer battle- one of
my best friends lost her mom 3 years ago, which was
something I had to watch/continue watching her
go through. I've lose 2 aunts to cancer as well. I'm
so happy for you that you were able to overcome
this disease and have been in remission for so
long. I hope you continue to live a long+healthy
life, and know that you aren't alone :)

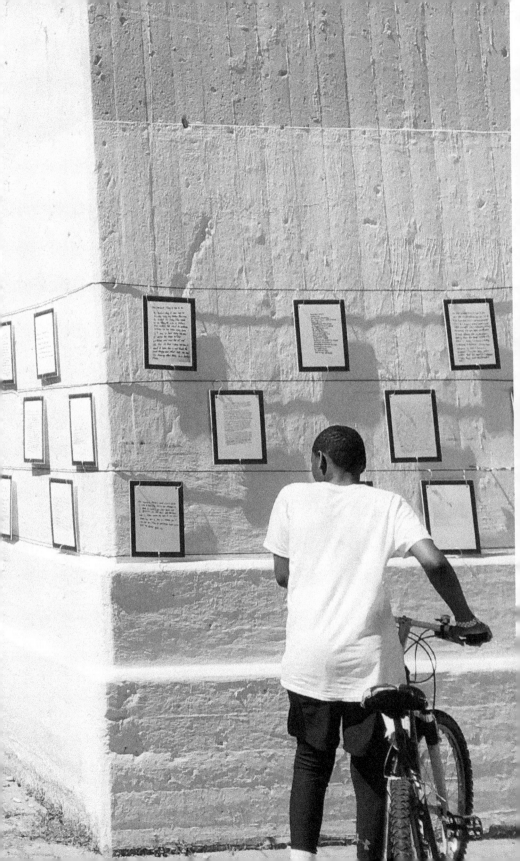

The Hardest thing I've ever had to do is,
Let my daughter go. She thinks shes grown and that she knows better for her life. she feels that my moth & sister wont do her wrong. she's only 17 with a baby. I haven't seen the two of them since february. So the best thing I could do is let her go and let GOD take controll of the whole situation.

To the person who wrote about
having to let her daughter go (17 yo with a baby)

As a mom of 3 kids, I can't
imagine how difficult this was for
you. But I also appreciate that sometimes
loving our kids the best is making those really
tough decisions on their behalf.
You are a good mom and yes, God
is ultimately in control. I am
praying for all of you — especially
your momma heart.

♡ xoxo

The hardest thing I've ever had to do..
believe that I was enough. By age
age nine I was living in my ninth
home with my grandpa because
my Mother died when I was six.

Foster Care will make you believe
no-body wants you. I guess
I still believe it's impossible for
someone to love me and I love
them. I just want to want up
and feel like I'm enough.

I want to love me
because I truly believe
I Am Enough. ♡

To the person who wrote about the challenge of believing they are enough — such a hard personal challenge but such an important result. I am so proud of you for digging deep and learning how to love yourself. Simply put — you are enough exactly how you are today. What you bring into this world is uniquely special. Keep your head high and remember everything you need is within you.

To the person that had a hard time believing that they were enough. I would like to tell you how much you mean to me. I want you to know that you are so brilliant and so magnificent in every way. You are perfect, and every second, every day, every week, every month, and every year that you spend in this world, is all worth it. The way that you smile, the way that you laugh, and the way that your eyes sparkle, make you incredibly precious. Please, never let anyone dampen that light within you that brightens the world. Above all else, know that you are infinitely loved, and no one will ever be able to change that.

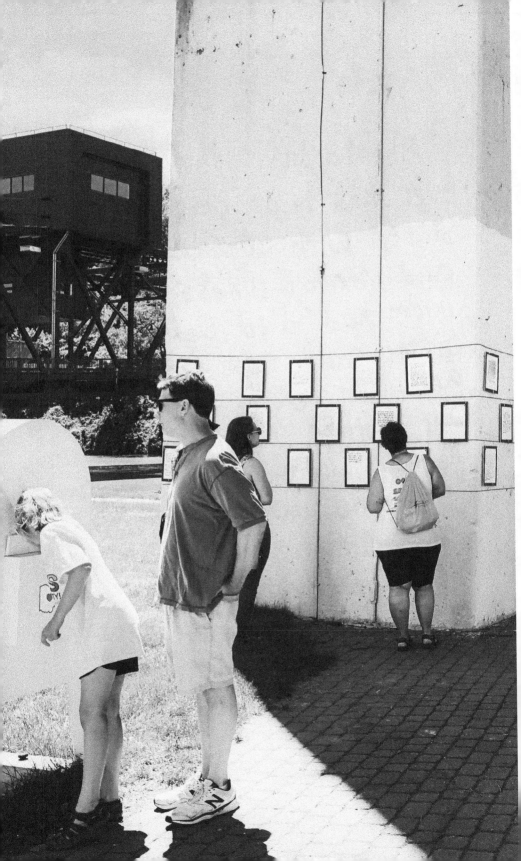

The hardest thing I ever had to do was tell my sister with cognitive disability and mental illness that our mom had died sudenly. My sister can't cope with change and was very codependent with our mother. My sister upon hearing the news, held my hand, asked questions cried and wanted ice cream. Sometimes my sister forgets my mam is gone. Other times she demands her ashes. It's never easy, but it's real and honest, just as mental illness is.

Dear Person who had to tell their mentally ill Sister that your mother has passed away. You have to know this letter right at me. I have never had to deal with anything along these lines. knowing someone like you and your story has put me back in perspective. I want you to know ppl like me are hear somewhere, to listen, to sympisize with You about these challenges. You are strong,

You are brave, keep getting through it you've came this far! Now, there is no turning back ♡ You will come out of this conquer this & you will be stronger than before. Just know pp, want to hear your story, Its inspirational, and shows how strong humans really are. You are strong — just never sive up! You got this!

The hardest thing I had to do was have my mom take me to the pych hospital for the second time because I tried to take my life for the third time

Call and tell my parents that I was being admitted to a psych hospital for suicidal Ideation.

To The Person who had to tell their parents that they needed to be admitted to a Pych hospital I feel really bad because when I went to tell my mom I needed - to go to therapy for suisidal prevention so I know its hard but it can only get better and as parents their job is to support + make the best you possible. I wish you the best of luck.

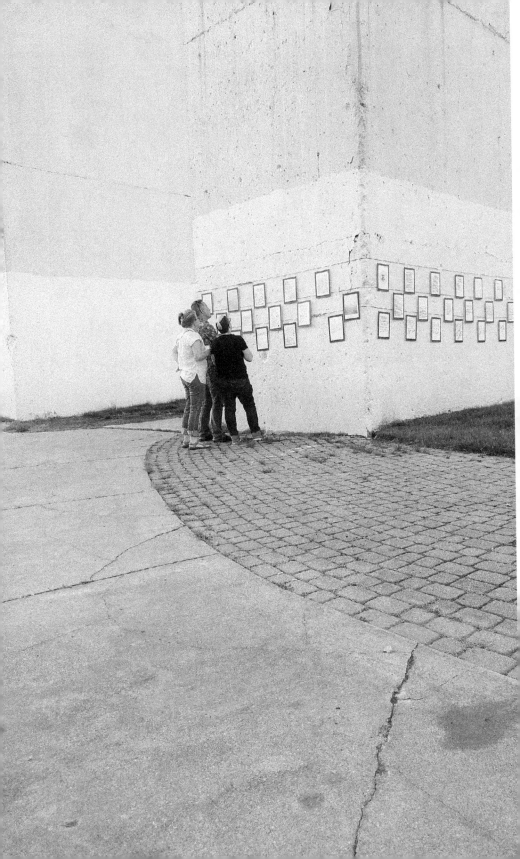

The hardest things I had to go
through was growing up as a deaf
and hard of hearing person. My
mother is spanish and do not know
any english. I can speak pretty
Clear. I speak now 3 lang.
I learn to overcome my weakness.
Be the best competition to yourself
and be come a better you!
Faith and attitude is the Key to
Success!

To the person who has a hearing struggle, you are awesome! I would never be able to make it and I appreciate how brave and strong you are! You are different! You are strong! You are brave! I am so proud of you! It takes gut sharing your private stories and your insecurities. I couldneve be able to do so! your courageousness gives me hope and strength to be proud about who I am, and now I am! you inspire many people! keep on going and living life! You are amazing!

The hardest thing I ever had to do was make my daughter cry.

When I left her dad she was seven years old and loved him with all her heart. She thought that holes in walls and bruises on her mommy were just scary things that sometimes happen to everyone. It shouldn't be that way.

I couldn't tell her we were moving. I couldn't risk her telling him. when I left, it took two hours. I only took her toys and our clothes. Ten years worth of my life and seven of hers got left behind. The house I bought, with everything in it, was abandoned. She was so scared; and mad. She yelled at me that it was my fault and that we needed to go back. It crushed me.

That was five years ago. This week she very casually told me she likes where we live, her stepdad, her life and that I should have left her dad sooner.

She has no idea how important that is to me.

To the person who saw
your daughter cry: Sometimes
doing the thing we have to do
hurts the people we love.
There is no good way around
that - there is only going through
it. And you kept going. How
lucky your daughter is to
have you, a mother who cares
so much, who is so resilient,
whose strength of spirit shines
through her words. you are
remarkable - and so is your
daughter. your story is
filled with hope.
♡

The hardest thing I've had to do is watch my vibrant Grandpa succumb to cancer. My whole life he was this warm, jolly constant in my life. Watching him deteriorate was excruciating. He went from the perpetual life of the party to a shell of himself so quickly. Watching him cry in pain was heart breaking. I don't choose to remember him that way. I'll always remember him smiling, laughing, joking and bringing every dance floor he stepped onto to life!

The hardest thing I've ever had to do was say goodbye to my grandpa for the last time. My mom picked me up from school and told me that he was dying. We sat in the lobby at school and called him on the phone. We sat on the phone with him as he was in the hospital. He sounded very sick and weak. I couldn't get words out because I was crying so I just listened to him tell me he loved me.

To the one who lost thier
grandfather, and others who
had loss.

I am old now. But I remember
when I had my first big loss,
my brother. It seemed like
the colors had left the world
like I was never going to
feel joy again. But gradually
you do feel better. Eventually
you will except that it is all
a part of being alive.
eventually you can have joy
and sorrow and gratitude
for everyday. Even the
tough ones

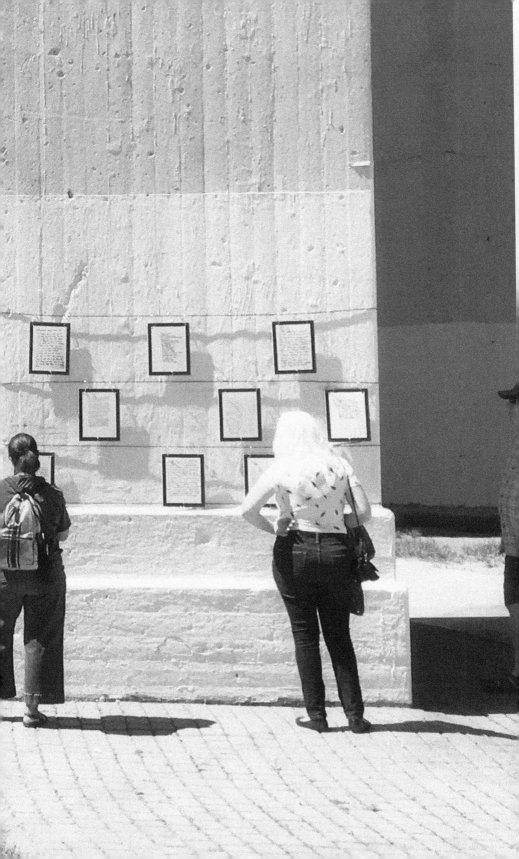

the hardest thing I've gone through is trying to lose weight. I've always dislike my body. But being in 7th grade makes it hard to lose weight. I cannot do diets and rarely ever have time to workout. I am still struggling with this. And going through this is an emotional rollercoaster. I cry because I feel hopeless. I cry because I feel lonely.

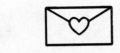

To the person who is trying to lose weight,

There is hope. If you feel that you aren't good enough, or thack others are being mean to you just because you don't look like them, just know this:

You are enough! It is horrible of others to treat you like that. You should feel bad for them that they have to bring you down, just to make ~~themselves~~ feel ~~good~~ better. If this important enough to you, you can accomplish anything! 7th grade will be over soon, but the best way to get through it is to love yourself.

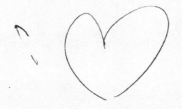

The hardest thing I've ever have to do was move away from my family for college. After college, I still continued to live away from home. Every day I think about my family and I cry often because I miss them so much. I've learned to value my family and cherish every moment I spend with them. I've found a home away from home in NE Ohio and I love it here. In August my family is going to visit me and I'm so excited to see them.

To the person who had a hard time leaving their family to go to college,

It is okay! Things will get better. Focus on the good: making new friends, trying new things, and looking forward to the bright path ahead of you! You know you are loved by your friends and family back home, and use that to make every day more special. Love and support are the best feelings in the world, and reflecting on this is a beautiful thing that helps you overcome challenges. I know this time may be hard right now, but looking back in your future years, college will be an unforgettable experience that sets a foundation for success. Your family and friends back hom want this for you! Just take on every new day thinking about their support, and smile ü. You are loved!

Everything will brighten up very soon.

The hardest thing i had to do, is cut a friend off from my life. This was one of my best friends, since middle school, but due to how the relationship turned into i felt it was one sided & unhealthy so i had to stop with it.

To the person who wrote that they had to cut off one of their best friends, I went through something very similar. My friend group was always very close and we had been like that for about 4 years. I never would have thought that one day we would be split, but we did. They were not treating me and other few girls right, leaving us out and not acting like real friends. This was so shocking to me because it came out of no where. For a while, I just would let it slide and pretend like nothing was wrong because I did not want to believe what was right in front of me. So, me and the other 4 girls who were being treated wrongly decided that we had to let our other friends go. This was especially hard for one of my friends because she had to leave her best friend of 5 years. Thinking about it makes me sad sometimes because of all the great memories we had together. But the other part of me is happier because I know we made the right choice. I know how hard cutting things off with your friends can be, but in the end, it sometimes needs to be done. I am so thankful now for my amazing friends and I have gained a new confidence and freedom. Just know that everything happens for a reason♥ stay positive ☺

The hardest thing I've ever had to do was pressing charges agianst my most recent ex. Domestic violence and telecommunication harassment is a real thing. I did not even realize it was happening because I was under the impression that it was all out of love. Acknowledging toxicity was my biggest challenge. Recognizing that I deserved better, that I was strong enough to leave was an internal battle. I was scared of what they were capable of doing, not only to me but the people around me. My support system was there for me, guiding me through my personal struggles of walking away. With my broken heart knowing someone could say they loved you could hurt you so badly was hard. The people around me reminded me I am strong. After I had the courage to leave it only made this person more upset. Where I was then stalked. Authorities were involved, and never in a million years did I think this would be the result. I am good now. I am strong.

To the person who had to press charges against their recent ex for domestic violence + telecommunications harassment: I applaud your courage, strength, resilience, and ability to move forward!
I was in a similar situation and I was so lucky to have support when I finally decided to walk away. I want to tell you → things DO get better! The pain does fade, and you will absolutely meet people who love you and treat you as you deserve to be treated! The hardest part is over.
I am so glad you had the courage to call the authorities, even though I know that was probably not easy! I ask all victims to trust that there really are people in law enforcement + other social services who really WANT to help! I became a police officer because I was a victim/survivor and I know how scary it is! There is hope and life after abuse. Take it seriously and ask for help. Everyone deserves peace in their home. ♡

Being able to forgive
my dad.

Hardest thing I ever had to do was walk away from my father. He wasn't ready to be a father and husband. He chose to be a husband first. I was 14 when I realized that. Im 33 now and still love my old bestfriend but now I feel better knowing Im happy to have other father figures. Peace  and blessings

The hardest thing I ever had to do was accept my biological father never wanted me or loved me. I spent many years feeling guilt that I was born. I had to attend years in counseling I was NOT the problem. He should have loved me and considered me a blessing. I accept that I do not love him. Everything I lost in him I found in other people.

To the people with not so great
fathers:

I'm sorry it sounds like your dad
is like mine. I don't understand
how you abandon a child. I don't
understand how you don't love your
child. But I'm happy I don't understand
because if I understood then I would
be like him and I'm so grateful
I'm not. I don't need him to love
me - I am free of all that. I hope
you all can be free of that weight
too. It's all on him. You are worthy
and wonderful people who deserved
to have a father that was there.
I'm sorry you didn't get what you
deserved.

The hardest thing I
ever had to do was
go to the penetentary.
Now I'm in a shelter
and I don't have any family.

I'm vaiting on a settlement
but it hasn7 come yet.
Now I live my life day
by day, hour by hour, and
~~Mitoe~~ minute by minute

To the person who is in a shelter and has no family.

I have so much hope for you and believe that with patience you will get a family. Everything needs time and that is okay. Try to not focus on what you can't change or have no control over, focus on you. This is your time for self discovery and time to figure out yourself before the universe gives you a family. Family can come in many different ways through friends and those who take time out of their day to spend with you. Have hope and be patient ♥. I know I have hope for you ☺

I went thow my dad pasing and I just went to a helping class with other kids that has someone that past and they helped me so ~~much~~ much.

To the person that wrote about their dad passing away and then going to a help group with other kids, I'm so sorry for your loss, but I'm happy that you found people like you to help with your grief. I have never experienced something like this, but I can't imagine what you went through. Surround yourself with positive people and try to keep a positive mindset even though I know it's hard. Let your emotions out and talk to people about it especially the kids like you. I hope you and your family are doing okay and I know you can get through these hard times.

For me it was making Friends in middle school cause I was alone for some of school cause I got double crossed by my best friend I made a new group of friend and some of my friends from 5th gread all forgot each other but now I have amizing friend and life is like a ocean theres somtimes waves and you got to get through them somtimes.

Dear person who had all your friends in elementary school, and lost them in middle School,

I totally understand how you feel. Don't ever loose hope! The right people will like you for you. You don't have to change anything about yourself to seem more interesting! you are plenty interesting! Things like this make you wonder what you did to deserve it, but sometimes you didn't do anything. Some people just don't like you because your strength reminds them of their weakness. People can be jealous of how good of a person you are. Stay true to you and believe in yourself!

. Don't let the world change your smile

let your smile change the world!

You Can!

The hardest thing I've ever had to do was admit to myself that something was wrong with me. I am an only child, and all through middle school, I did what I thought I was supposed to do. I got good grades, I played sports, I sang, I was student council president, and I expected myself to do it all, be the best at it, and be happy. I developed horrible anxiety which I told myself was just "pre-game jitters". These "jitters" were actually full panic attacks that could last hours. I would shake, I wouldn't be able to breathe, and when they got really bad, I thought it was best to distract myself. I dug my fingernails so deep into my wrists I would bleed. The worst part of it all was I hated myself for letting it happen. I finally broke down, and I was able to realize that how I reacted wasn't normal. I was putting huge amounts of pressure on myself and continuing to do things I didn't want to do just because I wanted to seem perfect.

I still have bad anxiety, but I see someone, and I'm learning how to let people in and stop blaming myself. I'm learning that if I need help it's not a burden because people want to help me.

To the person who wrote about anxiety and always trying to be perfect, you are not alone. I am here to cheer you on while you are out there doing the things you love because they are the activities that you want to do rather than the activities that you think you are expected to do. I hope you are proud of every accomplishment you achieve and every goal you reach. Be proud because you did your personal best. Be proud when you find the courage to ask others to join you on your walk through life. We would LOVE to help support you in any way we can. You show your strength when you ask for help so whenever you feel panicked, take a deep breath and continue to reach out to others.

To the person who wrote about having horrible anxiety and feeling the pressure to seem perfect, I am so glad that you are seeing someone and learning how to let people in, and to not blam yourself. I know how overwhelming the pressure to be perfect not only at school, but in your personal life as well can be. It is so important to be able to admit not only to yourself, but to other people as well that you need help, and finding a way to get help. I am constantly working to not blame myself for not feeling okay all the time. It is perfectly normal that when you need help you are getting help, and that it is not a burden, you are not a burden.

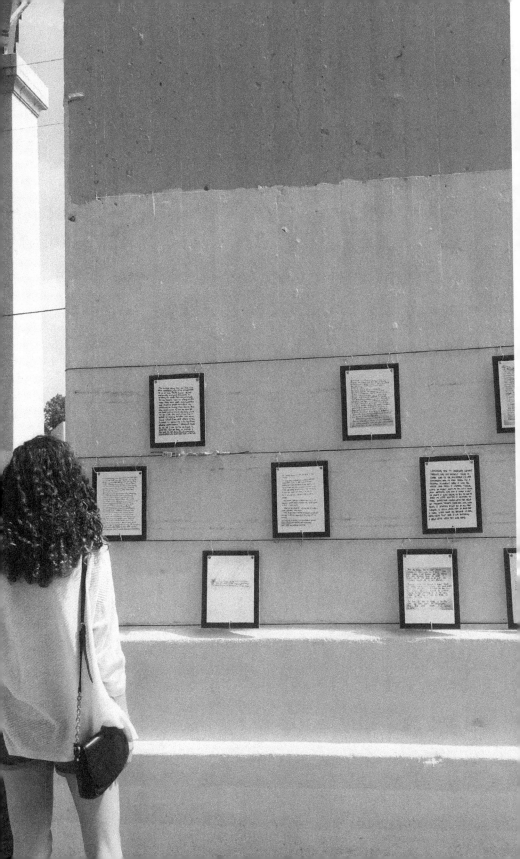

The hardest thing I have ever done was my sister battle breast cancer while being pregnant with my youngest nephew. At this time we also loss our grandmother. Watching my sister battle cancer truly broke me. Throughout this time my faith, morals, and values were being tested. So, how did I overcome this one might ask. I watched my sister keep her faith alive and push / preserve through such a difficult time. I knew if she could be strong, I had to be there & be strong for other and our family. I got closer with my faith / relationship with God and ask him to watch over us through this difficult time, and to alway give my sister the strength to preserve. My sister is now a 4 YEAR SURVIVOR & my nephew is 4 years old!

To the person who watched their sister
fight breast cancer while she was pregnant
with your nephew,

A few years ago my grandmother was diagnosed
with cancer and she like your sister survived.
However, I feel very guilty because I was
much younger and naive to her situation.
She had to be treated at a hospital in
Pittsburg and today looking back I
feel awful that I was not able to
be there for her every step of the
way. I love my grandma and like
you have learned to cherish the time
with the ones that I love. You
can't predict the future, only love and
spend time with the ones that mean
the most today. Thank you for your
strength and for your sister's strength.
I wish the best to you and
your family. God bless you.
  I need to go hug my sister now.

The hardest thing ive dealt with was getting help with my anxiety and my overall Mental Health. I relized that i needed help when I became rally negitive with everything. I would take out my anger on others once I got help ive been very harry. though times still get rough.

To the person who wrote about dealing with their mental health, your story was so inspiring & you are so strong for being able to fight through those obstacles. By sharing your story, I know you've inspired so many more people to be open to sharing their story or enabled them to not be afraid & to feel that they can do something to combat their difficult times. Going through these issues & being able to come out of it strong, amazes people. Dealing with mental illness is something that a lot of people aren't comfortable sharing or talking about & is something that not everyone can completely understand. Having to go through that type of thing with the way others feel can be hard, but having the strength to share your story & your experience is so amazing & inspiring.

Living In A Tent

For 5 months I lived in a Tent down by the West Bank Riverbed. This experience was truly a Life changing tramatic experience. I had to fight off the invasion of numerous Raccoons. Each day was a lesson in life as a homeless person. There were times when I couldn't Wash on days on End. Living Homeless in a Tent taught me the Value of Responsibility and how to be sustainable with my Responsibilities Today I am very grateful for those Lessons and now I live each day with purpose.

The hardest thing I ever had to do was to forgive myself for not visiting my grandmother in the hospital. the day she died. I had gotten breakfast with my friends that morning & I knew that my family was leaving to visit in the afternoon. Finishing breakfast, I knew I had enough time to drive back so that I could go visit her, but my friend asked if I was free so I said yes. We had been visiting my grandma each Saturday, so I figured I could see her next week since she didn't seem that weak. That night, my sister told me that my grandma just died. I couldn't help, but feel mad at myself for not visiting her that day. I told my father how I felt and he reminded me not to be so hard on myself &, to be grateful that I was able to see her the weekend before. I began to forgive myself as I went to her wake & funeral knowing that she wouldn't want me to be mad, but rather have me be grateful for the times I've had with her.

The hardest thing I have ever done is get divorced. Serving in the military in Iraq had its challenges. People got shot three times and I was either there when it happened or I was in the team collecting the wounded off of the street. Divorce was harder than my military experience because it felt like it was dangerous to those I love. I didn't have a perfect daughter to worry about in that desert heat. My daughter could easily have been a casualty of my divorce and that reality was never lost on me. Inertia, Faith, Logic. Call it what you want, but getting through that stretch seemed like the only option. Years later, my daughter remains perfect and I have found happiness. "Nothing lasts forever, and we both know hearts can change..."

The hardest thing I've had to do was
take care of my mother who had
stage 4 breast cancer. We took
care of her for 7 years and it
was difficult in all ways.
But in the end, when she died, I
realized that it was a gift to spend
more time with her and for her to
spend time with her grand babies.

The hardest thing I've ever had to do is look inwards.

The first time I realized how necessary and how painful that is I was 17, and I was in another country, and I was shrouded in my own apathy, and self-absorbtion, and anger, and when I looked at those things and started to shed them, it felt like picking a scab that wasn't quite ready — it was raw, and it hurt, and once I started I had to see it through.

I was outside, under this incredible night sky, in this beautiful Central American mountain, and I forced myself to do it. I asked myself,

"What are you afraid of?" And the fear of inadequacy, waste, unlovedness, rushed into me.

"What do you want?" And the not knowing rushed into me and so did the beginnings of being okay with not knowing.

It is easy not to do this — to stay inside of yourself forever to avoid pain and fear and uncertainty, but I refuse to, and I hope you do too.

The hardest thing I had to do was to go back to college and complete my degree after 27 yrs. I had 2 children at an early age and took time to raise them. After they became grown it was my turn to start anew. I jump in with both feet, scared, and unsure but I always believe I was worth it to better myself. So here I am at fabulous Fifty getting my degree in Social Work. Fearless!

IF you have shared the hardest thing you have ever had to do, you have taken a step. It may seem impossible, but we read your stories and may ache, but grow _hope_ in seeing how you survived and are persisting. You are okay and still here, among a community who cares and feels with you and for you. Whatever you may carry, you are not alone.

Never, ever give up.

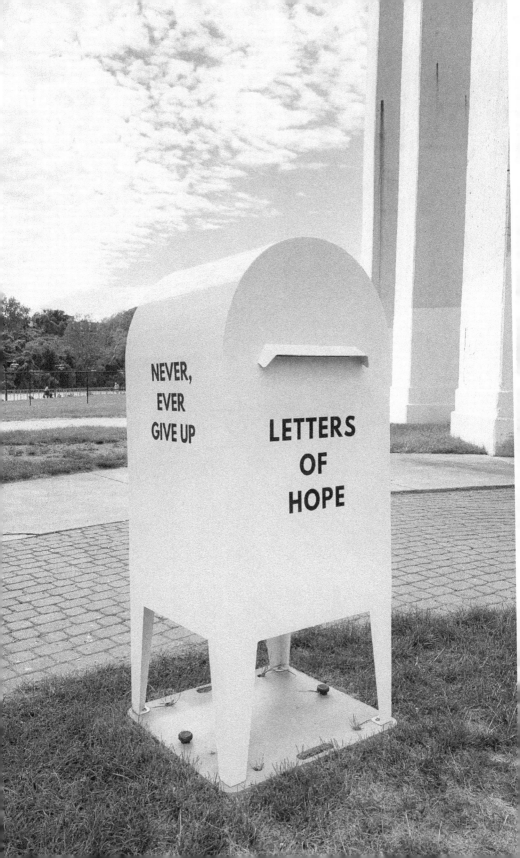